DEPRESSED TEENAGE CHILD.

A GUIDE ON IDENTIFYING DEPRESSION IN CHILDREN AND TEENAGERS, AND STRATEGIES TO HELP THEM RECOVER QUICKLY.

ELLIANA P. LEVI Ph.D.

TABLE OF CONTENTS.

into Treatment Plans

CHAPTER 6:

BUILDING RESILIENCE AND COPING SKILLS.

- Teaching Emotional Regulation Techniques

- Encouraging Healthy Lifestyle Habits

- Fostering Positive Relationships and Peer Support

CHAPTER 7:

ADDRESSING STIGMA AND MISCONCEPTIONS.

- Educating Communities about

Hobbies and Activities

- Exploring Opportunities for

Personal Growth

CHAPTER 10:

NURTURING HOPE AND RECOVERY.

- Celebrating Progress and

Small Victories

- Emphasizing the Importance

of Long-Term Support.

INTRODUCTION.

Welcome to the comprehensive guide on understanding and addressing depression in children and adolescents. In today's fast-paced and ever-changing world, the mental well-being of our youth is of utmost importance. As parents, caregivers, educators, and concerned individuals, it is crucial to recognize the signs of depression in young individuals and take proactive steps to support them through their challenging journey.

Chapter 1 delves into the intricate nature of childhood depression, shedding light on its manifestations across different age groups. By understanding the nuances of depression in youth, we can effectively identify warning signs and provide timely intervention.

In Chapter 2, we explore the multitude of factors that contribute to depression in children and adolescents. From biological influences to environmental stressors, gaining insight into these factors equips us with a deeper understanding of the complexities s urrounding youth mental health.

The pivotal role of parents and caregivers is highlighted in Chapter 3, emphasizing the importance of creating a nurturing and supportive environment at home. Effective communication and recognizing the need for professional help are essential components in guiding our youth through their struggles.

Chapter 4 addresses the process of seeking professional help, emphasizing the importance of identifying mental health professionals specialized in working with children and adolescents. We also navigate through accessing school-based support services to ensure a holistic approach to treatment.

In subsequent chapters, we delve into various treatment approaches for youth depression, building resilience and coping skills, addressing stigma and misconceptions, supporting academic success and social well-being, promoting a sense of purpose and fulfillment, and nurturing hope for recovery.

Join us on this insightful journey as we equip ourselves with the knowledge and tools to recognize, understand, and support our children and adolescents through their battle with depression.

Let's embark on this crucial exploration together, with the ultimate goal of fostering a supportive environment where our youth can thrive mentally, emotionally, and socially.

CHAPTER 1.

RECOGNIZING DEPRESSION IN CHILDREN AND TEENAGERS.

Childhood depression is a complex and intricate mental health condition that can have profound effects on a young person's emotional, social, and cognitive development. Understanding the intricate nature of childhood depression involves recognizing its multifaceted impact on various aspects of a child's life.

Firstly, childhood depression encompasses a wide range of emotional and behavioral symptoms that may differ from those seen in adults. Children may not always express their feelings of sadness directly; instead, they may exhibit irritability, clinginess, or physical complaints such as stomachaches or headaches. These typical symptoms can make it challenging for adults to recognize and address the underlying depression in children.

the interplay between genetic predisposition and environmental factors further complicates the understanding of childhood depression. While genetic factors can contribute to a child's susceptibility to depression, environmental stressors such as family conflicts, trauma, bullying, academic pressures, or social isolation can also play a significant role in triggering or exacerbating depressive symptoms.

Furthermore, the impact of childhood depression extends beyond emotional distress to affect a child's cognitive functioning and academic performance. Depressed children may experience difficulties concentrating in school, leading to academic challenges and potential long-term consequences on their educational attainment and future opportunities.

Socially, childhood depression can lead to withdrawal from peers, strained relationships with family members, and an overall sense of disconnection from their support network. These social implications can further perpetuate the cycle of depression and hinder the child's ability to seek help and support.

Moreover, the stigma surrounding mental health issues adds another layer of complexity to childhood depression. Misconceptions about childhood depression may lead to delayed diagnosis and intervention, resulting in prolonged suffering for the affected child.

Recognizing the intricate nature of childhood depression involves acknowledging its unique manifestations in young individuals, understanding the interplay of genetic and environmental factors, and addressing its far-reaching impact on gt , cognitive, and social domains.

Interplay of genetic and environmental factors in the case of childhood depression.

Childhood depression is influenced by a complex interplay of genetic and environmental factors. Genetics plays a significant role, with research suggesting that children with a family history of depression are more likely to experience it themselves. Specific genes related to neurotransmitter function and stress response are implicated.

However, environmental factors also play a crucial role. Adverse childhood experiences such as trauma, abuse, neglect, or chronic stress can significantly increase the risk of depression in children. Family dynamics, parental mental health, socioeconomic status, and peer relationships also contribute to the environmental influences on childhood depression.

Moreover, gene-environment interactions are important. For instance, certain genetic predispositions may increase susceptibility to depression when combined with adverse environmental factors, while protective factors such as supportive relationships or access to mental health resources can mitigate the risk.

Understanding the interplay between genetics and environment is essential for developing effective prevention and intervention strategies for childhood depression, including early identification, family support, and targeted therapies that address both biological and psychosocial factors.

SIGNS OF DEPRESSION IN CHILDREN ?

The symptoms and symptoms of depression in young children include adjustments within inside the manner they sense,suppose or behaves .

Children with depression may experience a range of emotions and thoughts that can manifest in various ways:

Children with depression may feel:

cranky

irritable

angry, sad

anxious

Feelings:

1. Crankiness, irritability, and anger:

Children with depression may have difficulty regulating their emotions, leading to frequent outbursts of frustration or anger.

2. Sadness: Persistent feelings of sadness or emptiness are common in children with depression, impacting their overall mood and outlook on life.

3. Anxiety: Many children with depression also experience symptoms of anxiety, including excessive worrying, nervousness, and fearfulness.

4. Feelings of worthlessness: They may believe that they are a bad person or inherently flawed, leading to low self-esteem and self-criticism.

5. Hopelessness: Children with depression may feel that their difficulties are insurmountable and that there is no way to improve their situation.

6. Loneliness: They may perceive themselves as unlovable or believe that no one cares about them, leading to feelings of isolation and loneliness.

Children with depression may think:

> that they are a bad person
>
> their difficulties are their own fault
>
> that terrible factors will manifest in them, and they will fear a lot
>
> that no one loves them

Thoughts:

1. Self-blame: Children with depression may attribute their difficulties to personal failings, believing that they are responsible for their own unhappiness.

2. Catastrophic thinking: They may have pessimistic thoughts about the future, expecting the worst possible outcomes

and feeling overwhelmed by worries and fears.

3. Lack of self-really well worth thought: Negative minds approximately themselves can also additionally lead young children with depression to a sense of not fit to be loved, or helped , or happiness about themselves may lead children with depression to feel undeserving of love, support, or happiness.

4. Social isolation: They may withdraw from social interactions and activities, believing that they are unworthy of companionship or fearing rejection from others.

It's essential to recognize these signs and symptoms in children with depression and provide them with the support and resources they need to cope and recover effectively.

Children with depression can also additionally behave **in an uncommon approach, such as:**

not wanting to do things they enjoy, such as see friends

being angry and impulsive

doing much less nicely well in the academy than they commonly do

not feeling hungry, or eating too much.

Why Children with depression may exhibit unusual behaviors due to the impact of their condition on their emotions, thoughts, and physical well-being:

1. Loss of interest in activities: Children with depression may lose interest in activities they once enjoyed, such as seeing friends, participating in hobbies, or engaging in extracurricular

activities. This loss of interest is often a result of the pervasive feelings of sadness, hopelessness, and low ene rgy associated with depression.

2. Irritability and impulsivity: Depression can manifest as irritability and impulsivity in children, leading to sudden outbursts of anger or frustration. These behaviors may be a coping mechanism for dealing with overwhelming emotions or a response to feelings of worthlessness or inadequacy.

3. Academic decline: Depression can significantly impact cognitive functioning, including concentration, memory, and problem-solving skills. As a result, children with depression may struggle academically, experiencing a decline in their performance at school compared

to their usual level of achievement.

4. Changes in appetite: Depression can disrupt eating patterns, leading to changes in appetite. Some children may experience a loss of appetite and have difficulty eating, while others may turn to food as a source of comfort, leading to overeating or binge eating. These changes in eating habits can further exacerbate feelings of guilt, shame, or self-bl ame associated with depression.

Overall, the unusual behaviors exhibited by children with depression are often a reflection of their internal struggles and the ways in which depression affects their emotions, thoughts, and physical well-being. It's crucial for caregivers, teachers, and healthcare professionals to recognize these signs and provide appropriate support and intervention to help children manage their depression effectively.

UNDERSTANDING DEPRESSION IN THE YOUTHS.

Depression in youth is a complex and nuanced mental health condition that presents unique challenges and considerations compared to depression in adults. Understanding the nuances of depression in youth involves recognizing the specific factors that influence its development, manifestation, and impact on young individuals.

One of the key nuances of depression in youth is the overlap with typical adolescent behavior and mood fluctuations. Adolescence is a period of significant emotional, physical, and social changes, making it challenging to distinguish between normal teenage angst and clinically significant depression. This can lead to under diagnosis or misinterpretation of depressive symptoms in young individuals

Moreover, the symptoms of depression in youth may manifest differently than in adults. While feelings of sadness and hopelessness are common across age groups, young people may also exhibit irritability, anger outbursts, academic decline, changes in sleep or eating patterns, social withdrawal, and risk-taking behaviors. These varied presentations require a nuanced understanding to accurately identify and address depression in youth.

The role of social media and digital technology is another important nuance in understanding depression in youth. The constant exposure to social media platforms, cyberbullying, comparison with idealized images online, and the pressure to curate a perfect online persona can contribute to feelings of inadequacy, isolation, and low self-esteem among young individuals. These factors can exacerbate depressive symptoms and complicate the management of depression in youth.

Family dynamics and relationships also play a crucial role in the development and course of depression in youth. Adverse childhood experiences, family conflicts, lack of parental support or supervision, insecure attachment styles, or a history of trauma can increase the risk of depression in young individuals. Addressing these familial factors is essential for effective prevention and intervention strategies.

Access to mental health resources and stigma surrounding mental illness are additional nuances that impact depression in youth. Limited awareness about mental health issues, reluctance to seek help due to fear of judgment or shame, financial barriers to treatment, and inadequate mental health services tailored to young individuals can hinder their ability to receive timely and appropriate care.

Understanding the nuances of depression in youth involves considering the interplay of developmental factors, symptom presentation, social influences, family dynamics, technological advancements, and access to mental health support. By recognizing these complexities, we can better support young individuals experiencing depression and promote their mental well-being.

The causes of depression in youth are multifaceted and influenced by various developmental, social, familial, and technological factors:

1. **Developmental factors:** Adolescence is a period of significant developmental changes, both biologically and psychologically.

Hormonal fluctuations, brain development, identity formation, and the challenges of transitioning to adulthood can all contribute to the onset of depression in youth.

2. **Symptom presentation:** Depression may present differently in youth compared to adults. While some symptoms, such as persistent sadness or loss of interest, are common across age groups, youth may also exhibit symptoms such as irritability, academic decline, social withdrawal, or reckless behavior. Understanding these variations in symptom presentation is crucial for accurate diagnosis and treatment.

3. **Social influences:** Social factors, including peer relationships, social media use, societal expectations, and academic pressure, can significantly impact the mental health of youth. Peer rejection, bullying, social isolation, or exposure to trauma can increase the

risk of depression in vulnerable individuals.

4. **Family dynamics:** Family environment and dynamics play a critical role in the development of youth depression. Factors such as parental conflict, parental mental health issues, substance abuse within the family, neglect, or abuse can contribute to feelings of insecurity, low self-esteem, and emotional distress in children and adolescents.

5. **Technological advancements:* * While technology offers numerous benefits, excessive use of digital devices, social media, and online platforms can also contribute to youth depression. Cyberbullying, comparison with idealized images on social media, sleep disruption due to screen time, and reduced face-to-face interactions can negatively impact mental health.

Understanding the interplay of these factors is essential for effective prevention and intervention strategies for youth depression. Early identification, supportive family and social environments, access to mental health resources, and promoting healthy coping mechanisms are crucial in addressing the complex causes of depression in youth and fostering resilience and well-being.

Signs and Symptoms of depression across different age groups.

The signs and symptoms of depression can vary across different age groups, reflecting the unique developmental stages and experiences of individuals. Here's an overview of the signs and symptoms of depression in various age groups:

Children and Pre-Adolescents (Up to 12 years old):

1. Irritability and mood swings

2. Social withdrawal or reluctance to engage in play or activities

3. Changes in appetite or weight

4. Complaints of physical symptoms such as stomachaches or headaches

5. Difficulty concentrating or declining academic performance

6. Feelings of worthlessness or guilt

7. Recurrent thoughts of death or suicide, although this may be expressed indirectly

Adolescents and Teenagers (13 to 18 years old):

1. Contentious, constant or Persistent feelings of sadness, hopelessness, or emptiness

2. Irritability, anger outbursts, or hostility

3. Loss of hobby in formerly lov ed activities

4. Changes in sleeping methods – inability to sleep or immoderate sleeping

5. Changes in appetite and noticeable

weight changes

6. Fatigue, lack of energy, or difficult to focus on something

7. Thoughts of death or suicide, expressed directly or indirectly

8. Risk-taking behaviors such as substance abuse, reckless driving, or self-harm

Adults (18 years old and above):

1. Persistent feelings of sadness, anxiety, or emptiness

2. Loss of interest in hobbies, work, or social activities

3. Changes in sleeping methodology – inability to sleep or immoderate sleeping

4. Appetite and weight changes

5. Fatigue, lack of energy, and decreased productivity

6. Feelings of worthlessness, guilt, or hopelessness

7. Difficultconscious focusing on

something, making choices or taking decisions, or remembering details

8. Recurrent thoughts of death or suicide

Elderly Adults (65 years old and above):

1. Persistent feelings of sadness, despair, or hopelessness

2. Social withdrawal and isolation from family and friends

3. Loss of interest in hobbies and activities previously enjoyed

4. Changes in appetite and weight loss

5. Sleep weakness - problems falling asleep or staying asleep

6. Aches and pains without a clear physical cause

7. Difficulty concentrating and making decisions

It's important to note that individuals may experience a combination of these symptoms to varying degrees, and not everyone will exhibit all the listed signs. Additionally, cultural factors, personal coping styles, and underlying medical conditions can influence how depression presents itself across different age groups.

How to distinguish depression from normal developmental challenges:

Understanding the Difference between Depression vs Normal Developmental Challenges

Growing up can be tough, and it's normal for young people to face challenges as they navigate through different stages of life. However, it's important to recognize when these challenges may be something more serious, like depression. Here are some ways to distinguish between the two:

1. Duration and Intensity Normal developmental challenges often come and go, causing temporary feelings of sadness or stress. However, if these

feelings persist for a long time (more than a couple of weeks) and are very intense, it could be a sign of depression.

2. Impact on Daily Life

While facing developmental challenges, young people may still be able to engage in their daily activities and hobbies. In contrast, depression can significantly disrupt their ability to function normally, affecting their schoolwork, relationships, and overall well-being.

3. Physical Symptoms

Depression can manifest in physical symptoms such as changes in appetite, sleep disturbances, and unexplained aches and pains. These physical signs are less common in normal developmental challenges.

4. Self-Esteem and Self-Image

Feeling unsure about oneself is a common part of growing up. However, if a young person consistently has extremely negative thoughts about themselves and a persistent sense of worthlessness, it may indicate depression rather than just normal self-doubt.

5. Social Withdrawal

While it's normal for young people to occasionally want some alone time or feel shy in social situations, persistent withdrawal from friends and family without any interest in activities they used to enjoy could be a sign of depression.

6. Suicidal Thoughts

Any point or trace of suicidal mind or thought must continually be taken very significantly seriously as it is not a regular part of an adolescent or child's development and should always be taken seriously and is not a normal part of adolescent development.

It is essential for parents, teachers,

and caregivers to be aware of these differences so they can provide the necessary support and seek professional help if needed.

By understanding these distinctions, we can better support young people as they navigate through the ups and downs of growing up.

CHAPTER 2.

FACTORS CONTRIBUTING TO DEPRESSION IN YOUTHS AND CHILDREN.

Understanding What Causes Depression in Young People Especially Children.

Depression is a serious issue that can affect young people, and it can be caused by many different things. Let's take a look at some of the reasons why young people might become depressed.

1. Feeling Sad for a Long Time

Sometimes, young people especially Children, feel sad or down for a long time, and this can lead to depression. It's important that parents, caregivers or guardians observe and to talk about these feelings so to get help them in time and when needed.

2. Tough Things Happening

When tough things happen, like someone passing away, parents separating, or other big changes, it can make young people feel really sad and lonely. These tough events can contribute to depression.

3. Feeling Bad About Themselves

Some young people might feel really bad about themselves, thinking they're not good enough or that nobody likes them. These thoughts can make them feel even worse and contribute to depression.

4. Family and Friends

Sometimes, problems within the family or with friends can make young people feel very stressed and unhappy. This stress can make them more likely to become depressed.

5. Feeling Pressured

Young people often feel pressure to do well in school or in activities they're involved in. This pressure can be overwhelming and lead to feelings of sadness and hopelessness.

6. Things They Do

Certain things they do like   - Substance abuse, Experimentation with drugs or alcohol can exacerbate depressive symptoms in adolescents.

7. spending too much time on screens can make young people more likely to become depressed. It's important for them to have healthy habits and activities.

8. Feeling Left Out

When young people feel left out or bullied by others, it can make them feel really alone and sad. This feeling of being left out can contribute to depres sion

9.Psychological Factors:

- Low self-esteem: Negative self-perception and feelings of inadequacy can contribute to the development of depression.

- Stressful life events: Traumatic

experiences, such as loss of a loved one, abuse, or significant life changes, can trigger depressive symptoms.

- Co-occurring mental health conditions: Conditions like anxiety disorders or attention-deficit/hyperactivity disorder (ADHD) can increase the risk of depression in children and adolescents.

10. Cultural and Societal Influences:

- Stigma around mental health: Negative attitudes toward seeking help for mental health issues can prevent children and adolescents from accessing support.

- Socioeconomic factors: Limited access to resources, unstable living conditions, or exposure to community violence can contribute to the development of depression.

It's important for young people to know that they're not alone and that there are ways to get help when they're feeling this way.

By understanding these different reasons for depression, we can work together to support young people who are going through a tough time.

Contributing to Depression in Children and the Youth":

Depression in children and adolescents can be influenced by a multitude of factors, encompassing biological, psychological, social, and environmental aspects. Here are several key contributors to depression in these age groups:

1. Biological Factors:

   - Genetic predisposition: Children and adolescents with a family history of depression or other mood disorders may have a higher risk of developing depression.

   - Neurochemical imbalances:

Imbalances in neurotransmitters such as serotonin and dopamine can play a role in the development of depression.

2. Social and Environmental Factors:

- Family dynamics: Conflict within the family, parental separation or divorce, or inadequate support from caregivers can impact a child's emotional well-being.

- Peer relationships: Bullying, social isolation, or peer rejection can contribute to feelings of loneliness and worthlessness.

- Academic pressure: High academic expectations and performance-related stress can be a contributing factor to depression in adolescents.

3. Lifestyle Factors:

- Substance abuse: Experimentation with drugs or alcohol can exacerbate depressive symptoms in adolescents.

- Sedentary lifestyle: Lack of physical

activity and excessive screen time may contribute to feelings of isolation and reduced well-being.

4. It's important to recognize that these factors interact and influence each other in complex ways. Additionally, individual experiences and resilience play a significant role in how these factors impact a child's or adolescent's mental health.

Understanding these diverse contributors is crucial for identifying and addressing the unique needs of children and adolescents experiencing depression.

CHAPTER 3.
THE ROLE OF PARENTS AND CAREGIVER.

The Role of Parents and Caregivers in Combating Depression in Children and Adolescents

Depression can significantly impact the lives of children and adolescents, affecting their emotional well-being, academic performance, and overall development. As parents and caregivers, your role in recognizing, addressing, and combating depression in young people is essential. Here are key aspects of your role in supporting children and adolescents facing depression:

1. Understanding Depression

Educating yourself about the signs, symptoms, and causes of depression in children and adolescents is crucial.

Awareness enables you to recognize potential indicators of depression early on.

Areas you as a parent or caregiver should pay more or close attention

To for early dictation of depression in your child's life as both children from 6 to 14 years because of their inabilities to understand or express their feelings.

Detecting depression in children and adolescents can be challenging, but parents and caregivers can watch for these signs:

1. **Changes in Behavior:** Look for sudden shifts in behavior, such as withdrawal from friends and family, irritability, or increased sensitivity.

2. **Emotional Changes:** Pay attention to mood swings, persistent sadness, or expressions of hopelessness.

3. **Changes in Sleep Patterns:* *

Notice if there are disruptions in sleep, such as insomnia or oversleeping.

4. **Changes in Appetite or Weight:* * Be aware of significant changes in eat ing habits or weight gain/loss.

5. **Loss of Interest:** If the child or adolescent loses interest in activities they once enjoyed, it could be a sign of depression.

6. **Physical Symptoms:** Watch for unexplained headaches or stomachaches that don't have a clear medical cause.

7. **School Performance:** Declines in academic performance, difficulty concentrating, or frequent absences may indicate underlying issues.

8. **Self-Harm:** Be alert to signs of self-harm, such as cuts or bruises, and take them seriously.

9. **Substance Use:** Increased use of drugs or alcohol can be a coping

mechanism for underlying depression which is in adolescents or youths.

10. **Expressed Thoughts of Self-Harm or Suicide:** Any mention of self-harm or suicide should be taken seriously and addressed immediately.

Regular communication with children and adolescents, and creating a friendly environment, are crucial steps in early detection and intervention. The most problem somechildren face in their homes is a problem of hostile and nagging environment, their parents are always hostile and abusive towards them so when they encounter any problems they should share with their parents or caregiver, they are terribly afraid of the negative outcome or reactions from them, and instead of talking to their parents or caregivers , they decides to bear it alone.

Some of them when try solving it themselves , they ends up being frustrated the more.

2. Creating a Supportive Environment

Fostering a supportive and nurturing environment at home where open communication is encouraged can help children and adolescents feel comfortable expressing their emotions and seeking help when needed.

When I see the way some parents embarrass their children, shun them and disregard their opinions in the home I feel so sad because most of those parents don't know that such actions create depression in children and adolescents, this is why many adolescents resort to alcohol and drugs in orders to find peace of the mind while many others thought finishing it up in suicide is theexceptional decision.

Parents must have to learn to give room for open communication in their homes in order to allow their children and adolescents communicate freely with them.

Sometimes as a parent or caregiver, seek the opinion of your child or children in certain issues that doesn't mean you are going to act on their opinions but to make them feel belonged especially in the areas of food to prepare school affairs and kind of clothes they will want you to buy for them, this act will open up their communication channels and make them feel belonged and love by their parents.

3. Active Listening and Validation

Actively listening to young people's concerns without judgment and validating their emotions can provide a sense of understanding and support, which is vital in combating feelings of isolation and hopelessness associated with depression.

Many instances dad and mom fail this listening aspect, you are expected to give attention to the reports or complaints your young children and adolescents lay before you or to you regarding academic environment, fellow baby bullying and teacher's hostility in the direction of them, manhandling of their caregivers and the molestation of their home lessons teacher.

Don't always be in a hurry they maybe trying to communicate something so important to you concerning these aforementioned areas above and the earlier you listen to them the better for the life of that child.

4. Encouraging Professional Help

Recognizing the importance of seeking professional help when dealing with depression is crucial. Encouraging young people to speak with mental health professionals, such as therapists or counselors, can provide them with the necessary support and interventions.

As we all know that every health aspect of a person's health challenge today has a professional or specialist in that area, so every patient or caregiver nee to have one or two for their family especially for the children and adolescent.

I seeking for a professional please note that he or she must be a child friendly professional not the rigid and source type that will end up complicating the whole situation.

5.   Promoting   Healthy   Coping Mechanisms

Teaching children and adolescents healthy coping strategies to manage stress, anxiety, and depressive symptoms is essential. Encouraging activities such as physical exercise, creative outlets, or mindfulness practices can contribute to their emotional well-being.

These are some of the healthy coping strategies for the children and adolescent to save them from depression.

Sure, here's an outline of various coping strategies for children and adolescents to manage stress, anxiety, and depressive symptoms, including different types of sports:

I. Mindfulness and Relaxation Techniques

   A. Deep breathing exercises

   B. Progressive muscle relaxation

   C. Guided imagery

   D. Mindful meditation

II. Physical Activity and Sports

   A. Team Sports

      1. Soccer

    2. Basketball

    3. Volleyball

  B. Individual Sports

    1. Swimming

    2. Tennis

    3. Martial arts

  C. Outdoor Activities

    1. Hiking

    2. Cycling

    3. Skateboarding

III. Creative Outlets

  A. Art therapy

  B. Music therapy

  C. Writing/journaling

IV. Social Support

  A. Spending time with friends and

family

B. Joining clubs or groups with similar interests

V. Healthy Lifestyle Habits

A. Balanced diet

B. Sufficient sleep

C. Limiting screen time

VI. Seeking Professional Help

A. Therapy (e.g., cognitive-behavioral therapy)

B. Counseling

C. Support groups

Each of these strategies can be adapted to suit the preferences and needs of individual children and adolescents, providing them with a variety of tools to manage their mental health effectively.

6. Monitoring Screen Time and Social Media Use

Being mindful of the impact of excessive screen time and social media use on young people's mental health is important. Setting boundaries and promoting healthy technology use can help mitigate potential negative effects on their well-being.

Cyber bullying among teenagers has gotten to an alarming stage, you as a parent or caregiver must be watchful of the activities your child or children are engaging in in social media to avoid becoming depressed as a result of social media bullying.

You must set boundaries and time limit for social media activities in your home especially for the children and adolescents ones, as this will help you ascertain the mental state of your child and know when depression is building up in them.

In setting up boundaries and time limit, you must do it in love and care to avoid your child seeing you as the enemy of their joy and happiness

7. Modeling Self-Care Practices

Demonstrating healthy self-care practices such as managing stress effectively, seeking support when needed, and maintaining a balanced lifestyle can serve as a positive example for young people.

As a parent or caregiver, you must lead by example as there is this general belief that children learn fast by what they see with their eyes than what they are thought.

So you must model yourself in your children especially when there is a challenge that can lead to depression in your own end, the children will always see your reaction and approach towards recovery and then learn. This is why you must have to show them a strength and courage.

8. Advocating for Comprehensive Support

Advocating for comprehensive support within the community, including access to mental health services in schools or local organizations, can contribute to a supportive network for young people struggling with depression.

As parents or caregivers, you must know that the mental health of your or a child is very important aspect that needs daily attention, check out your child to know if they are experiencing memory loss at some point, lack of comprehension, forgetfulness, and absent-mindedness. Finding out Earl enough can help you remedy the situation when it has not gotten to a chronic state.

As parents and caregivers, your active involvement in recognizing, addressing, and combating depression in children and adolescents plays a vital role in supporting their mental health and overall well-being.

Practical steps parents and caregivers are expected to take

Creating a Supportive Environment at Home:

1. Open Communication: Foster an environment where open, honest communication is encouraged. Make time for regular family discussions where everyone has the opportunity to express their thoughts and feelings in a non-judgmental setting.

2. Emotional Validation: Show empathy and understanding towards your children's emotions. Let them know that it's okay to feel sad, anxious, or upset, and reassure them that they can

always confide in you without fear of being dismissed or invalidated.

3. Establishing Routines: Consistent routines can provide a sense of stability and security for children and adolescents. Establishing regular meal times, bedtimes, and family activities can create a predictable and comforting environment.

4. Safe Space for Expression: Create a designated space within the home where children and adolescents can engage in activities that promote self-expression, such as art, writing, or music. This space can serve as an outlet for them to process their emotions.

Effective Communication with Children and Adolescents:

1. Active Listening: Practice active listening by giving your full attention when your children are speaking. Avoid interrupting and show genuine interest in what they have to say.

2. Non-verbal Cues: Pay attention to non-verbal cues such as body language and facial expressions. Sometimes, children may express their emotions through non-verbal means, and being attuned to these cues can help you understand their feelings better.

3. Encouraging Expression: Encourage your children to express their thoughts and feelings openly by asking open-ended questions and providing a safe space for them to share without fear of judgment.

4. Empathetic Responses: Respond empathetically to your children's

emotions. Let them know that their feelings are valid and offer support without dismissing or minimizing their experiences.

Recognizing the Need for Professional Help in the Journey of Combating Depression in Children and Adolescents:

1. Educate Yourself: Learn about the signs and symptoms of depression in children and adolescents so that you can recognize when professional help may be necessary.

2. Observing Behavioral Changes: Pay attention to significant changes in your child's behavior, such as withdrawal from social activities, changes in sleep patterns, or persistent irritability. These may indicate the need for professional intervention.

3. Seeking Professional Guidance: If you notice concerning signs of depression in your child or adolescent, it's important to seek professional help from a qualified mental health professional, such as a therapist or counselor.

4. Collaborative Approach: Work collaboratively with mental health professionals to ensure that your child receives comprehensive support tailored to their specific needs. This may involve therapy, counseling, or other evidence-based interventions.

By implementing these practical steps, parents and caregivers can contribute to creating a supportive environment at home, fostering effective communication with children and adolescents, and recognizing the need for professional help in combating depression in young people.

CHAPTER 4.
SEEKING PROFESSIONAL HELP.

Mental health is a vital aspect of a child or adolescent's overall well-being. However, when challenges arise, seeking professional help becomes essential. This chapter delves into the various aspects of seeking professional assistance for children and adolescents, including identifying mental health professionals, accessing school-based support services, and navigating the process of diagnosis and treatment.

Identifying Mental Health Professionals for Children and Adolescents

Finding the right mental health professional for a child or adolescent can be a daunting task for parents or caregivers. However, it's crucial to identify professionals who specialize in working with young individuals to ensure appropriate care and support. Some key professionals to consider include child psychologists, child psychiatrists, pediatricians with expertise in mental health, and licensed clinical social workers specializing in child and adolescent therapy.

Here are different duties of child psychologists, child psychiatrists, and pediatricians regarding children's health:

Child Psychologists:

1. **Assessment and Diagnosis:* * Child psychologists assess and diagnose various mental health conditions and developmental disorders in children and adolescents through interviews, observations, and standardized testing.

2. **Therapy and Counseling:** They provide psychotherapy and counseling services tailored to the unique needs of children and adolescents, addressing issues such as anxiety, depression, b ehavioral problems, and trauma.

3. **Behavioral Intervention:** Child psychologists develop and implement behavioral intervention plans to address behavioral challenges and promote positive coping strategies and adaptive behaviors.

4. **Parent and Caregiver Support:* * They offer guidance and support to parents and caregivers, helping them understand their child's behavior and develop effective parenting strategies to promote healthy development and well-being.

5. **Consultation:** Child psychologists often consult with other professionals, such as educators, pediatricians, and social workers, to

coordinate care and support for children with complex needs.

Child Psychiatrists:

1. **Diagnostic Evaluation:** Child psychiatrists conduct comprehensive diagnostic evaluations to assess children and adolescents for mental health disorders, including mood disorders, anxiety disorders, attention-deficit/hyperactivity disorder (ADHD), and autism spectrum disorders.

2. **Medication Management:** They prescribe and monitor medications to treat mental health conditions in children and adolescents, adjusting dosages and treatment plans as needed to optimize effectiveness and minimize side effects.

3. **Collaboration with Therapists:** Child psychiatrists collaborate with other mental health professionals, such as psychologists, counselors, and therapists, to develop integrated

treatment plans that address both the biological and psychosocial aspects of a child's mental health.

4. **Crisis Intervention:** Child psychiatrists provide crisis intervention services for children and adolescents experiencing acute mental health crises, such as suicidal ideation, self-harm, or psychotic episodes, to stabilize symptoms and ensure safety.

5. **Education and Advocacy:** They educate parents, caregivers, and the community about mental health issues affecting children and advocate for policies and resources that support early intervention and access to mental health care for children and adolescents.

Pediatricians:

1. **Well-Child Care:** Pediatricians provide routine well-child care, including physical examinations, immunizations,

and developmental screenings, to monitor children's growth and development and detect any p otential health concerns early.

2. **Early Intervention:** They identify and address developmental delays, behavioral concerns, and other health issues in children and adolescents through early intervention and referral to appropriate specialists or services.

3. **Health Promotion and Education:** Pediatricians educate parents and caregivers about child health and safety topics, such as nutrition, exercise, injury prevention, and sleep hygiene, to promote healthy lifestyles and prevent illness and injury.

4. **Management of Common Illnesses:** They diagnose and treat common childhood illnesses and injuries, such as colds, ear infections, asthma, and minor injuries, providing appropriate medical care and guidance

for recovery.

5.   **Coordination of Care:** * Pediatricians collaborate with other healthcare providers, educators, and community resources to coordinate comprehensive care and support for children and adolescents, ensuring continuity of care across different settings. When seeking a mental health professional, it's essential to consider factors such as their experience working with children and adolescents, their approach to therapy, and their availability. Additionally, seeking recommendations from trusted sources, such as pediatricians, school counselors, or other parents, can help narrow down the options and find a suitable match for the child's needs.

Accessing School-Based Support Services

Schools play a vital role in supporting

the mental health needs of children and adolescents. Many schools offer a range of support services aimed at addressing various mental health challenges that students may face. These services may include counseling programs, support groups, and interventions designed to promote men tal wellness.

Parents and caregivers can access school-based support services by reaching out to school counselors or mental health professionals employed by the school. These professionals can provide guidance on available resources and help coordinate support for students in need. Additionally, collaborating with school staff can help ensure continuity of care between home and school environments, facilitating a holistic approach to addressing mental health concerns.

Navigating the Process of Diagnosi s and Treatment

Navigating the process of diagnosis and treatment for mental health issues in children and adolescents can be complex and overwhelming. It often involves multiple steps, including assessment, diagnosis, treatment planning, and ongoing monitoring. Parents and caregivers play a crucial role in advocating for their child's needs and navigating the healthcare system to access appropriate care.

The process typically begins with an initial assessment conducted by a mental health professional to evaluate the child's symptoms and determine the need for further evaluation. This may involve standardized assessments, interviews, and observations to gather information about the child's behavior, emotions, and functioning. Based on the assessment findings, a diagnosis may be made, and a treatment plan tailored to the child's specific needs can be developed.

Treatment options may vary depending on the nature and severity of the child's mental health concerns but may include therapy, medication, or a combination of both. It's essential for parents and caregivers to actively participate in the treatment process, collaborate with mental health professionals, and advocate for their child's well-being every step of the way.

6 Major reasons why parents and caregivers must have to engage the service of child health professionals in handling or managing a depressed Child or adolescent.

Parents and caregivers must seek professionals to handle or manage a mentally depressed child or adolescent for several crucial reasons:

1. **Specialized Expertise:** Mental health professionals, such as child psychologists, child psychiatrists, and

licensed therapists, possess specialized training and expertise in assessing, diagnosing, and treating mental health disorders in children and adolescents. They are equipped with the knowledge and skills to identify the specific symptoms and underlying factors contributing to depression in young individuals.

2. **Accurate Diagnosis:** Depression in children and adolescents can manifest differently than in adults and may be mistaken for other issues or dismissed as typical teenage behavior. Mental health professionals can conduct comprehensive evaluations to accurately diagnose depression and differentiate it from other emotional or behavioral concerns. A precise diagnosis is essential for developing an appropriate treatment plan tailored to the child's needs.

3. **Individualized Treatment:* * Mental health professionals can provide

individualized treatment approaches tailored to the unique needs and circumstances of the child or adolescent. This may include various therapeutic modalities, such as cognitive-behavioral therapy (CBT), dialectical behavior therapy (DBT), play therapy, or family therapy, designed to address the underlying factors contributing to depression and promote healing and resilience.

4. **Medication Management:** In some cases, medication may be necessary to alleviate severe symptoms of depression or co-occurring mental health conditions in children and adolescents. Child psychiatrists can prescribe and monitor psychotropic medications, such as antidepressants or mood stabilizers, when indicated, carefully considering the child's age, developmental stage, and in dividual response to treatment.

5. **Safety and Crisis Intervention:* *

Mental health professionals can provide crucial support and intervention in situations where a depressed child or adolescent is at risk of self-harm, suicidal ideation, or other dangerous behaviors. They can implement safety plans, crisis interventions, and hospitalizations as needed to ensure the child's safety and stabilize their mental health symptoms.

6. **Support for Parents and Caregivers :** Parenting a child or adolescent with depression can be overwhelming and emotionally challenging. Mental health professionals not only provide support and guidance to the child but also offer education, coping strategies, and emotional support to parents and caregivers. They can help caregivers navigate the complexities of managing their child's depression, reduce feelings of guilt or inadequacy, and strengthen family communication and resilience.

In summary, seeking professional help

for a mentally depressed child or adolescent is essential to ensure accurate diagnosis, individualized treatment, safety, and support for both the young individual and their caregivers. Mental health professionals play a critical role in promoting healing, resilience, and improved quality of life for children and adolescents struggling with depression.

In conclusion, seeking professional help for children and adolescents experiencing mental health challenges as a result of unnoticed or prolonged depression is essential for promoting their overall well-being and resilience. By identifying appropriate mental health professionals, accessing school-based support services, and navigating the process of diagnosis and treatment, parents and caregivers can ensure that their child receives the care and support they need to thrive.

CHAPTER 5
TREATMENT APROACHES FOR YOUTHS AND CHILDREN DEPRESSION.

Depression in children and adolescents is a serious mental health concern that requires careful and comprehensive treatment approaches. This chapter explores various therapeutic modalities, medication considerations, and the integration of family therapy into treatment plans to address youth depression effectively.

Therapy and Counseling for Children and Adolescents

Therapy and counseling play pivotal roles in addressing youth depression by providing a safe space for children and adolescents to express their thoughts and feelings. Cognitive-behavioral therapy (CBT) has shown efficacy in treating youth depression by helping individuals identify and change negative thought patterns and behaviors. Play therapy is another valuable approach, especially for younger children, as it allows them to communicate and process emotions through play activities. Additionally, interpersonal therapy (IPT) focuses on improving relationships and communication skills, which can be particularly beneficial for adolescents struggling with interpersonal issues.

Medication Considerations and Alternatives:

While therapy is often the first line of treatment for youth depression, medication may be considered in cases of moderate to severe depression or when therapy alone is insufficient. Selective serotonin reuptake inhibitors (SSRIs) are commonly prescribed antidepressants for adolescents, although careful monitoring for potential side effects is essential. Other medication options, such as serotonin-norepinephrine reuptake inhibitors (SNRIs) or atypical antidepressants, may also be considered based on individual needs and response to treatment. However, it's crucial to weigh the potential benefits against the risks and involve parents or guardians in the decision-making process.

Incorporating Family Therapy into Treatment Plans:

Family therapy recognizes the interconnectedness of family dynamics and their impact on youth mental health. By involving family members in the treatment process, therapists can address underlying family conflicts, improve communication patterns, and foster a supportive environment for the young individual. Family therapy sessions may focus on enhancing parenting skills, resolving conflicts, and strengthening family relationships, all of which contribute to the overall well-being of the child or adolescent. Additionally, family therapy provides an opportunity for parents and caregivers to gain insight into their child's experiences and learn effective strategies for supporting their ment al health.

Conclusion:

Effective treatment approaches for youth depression encompass a combination of therapy, medication when necessary, and family involvement. By addressing the unique needs of each young individual within the context of their family environment, clinicians can help alleviate symptoms of depression and promote long-term mental health and resilience. Ongoing monitoring and collaboration between mental health professionals, families, and other support systems are essential to ensure comprehensive and holistic care for children and adolescents struggling with depression.

CHAPTER 6.
BUILDING RESILIENCE AND COPING SKILLS

Depression can significantly impact the lives of children and adolescents, affecting their emotional well-being, academic performance, and social interactions. Building resilience and coping skills is essential for helping young individuals navigate through depression and embark on a journey towards healing and recovery. In this chapter, we will explore how teaching emotional regulation techniques, encouraging healthy lifestyle habits, and fostering positive relationships and peer support can contribute to the healing process for children and adolescents dealing with depression.

Teaching Emotional Regulation Techniques:

Emotional regulation techniques are valuable tools for managing overwhelming emotions and reducing the symptoms of depression. Children and adolescents can benefit from learning various strategies to identify, express, and regulate their feelings in healthy ways. These techniques may include deep breathing exercises, mindfulness meditation, journaling, and progressive muscle relaxation.

Educating young individuals about the connection between thoughts, emotions, and behaviors can empower them to challenge negative thinking patterns and develop more adaptive coping strategies. By teaching emotional regulation techniques, children and adolescents can gain greater control over their emotions and build resilience in the face of depressive symptoms.

Encouraging Healthy Lifestyle Habits:

Healthy lifestyle habits play a crucial role in promoting overall well-being and resilience, especially for individuals struggling with depression. Encouraging children and adolescents to prioritize activities such as regular exercise, balanced nutrition, adequate sleep, and meaningful hobbies can have a positive impact on their mood and mental health.

Physical activity, in particular, has been shown to be effective in reducing symptoms of depression by releasing endorphins and improving brain function. By engaging in regular exercise, young individuals can boost their mood, reduce stress, and increase their resilience to depressive symptoms. Additionally, maintaining a nutritious diet and getting enough sleep are essential for supporting brain h ealth and emotional regulation.

Fostering Positive Relationships and Peer Support:

Positive relationships and peer support are vital sources of comfort, validation, and encouragement for children and adolescents experiencing depression. Fostering connections with caring adults, such as parents, teachers, counselors, and mentors, can provide young individuals with a sense of safety and security during difficult times.

Moreover, peer support groups and social activities can offer opportunities for young individuals to connect with others who may be experiencing similar challenges. Sharing experiences, offering mutual support, and building friendships can help reduce feelings of isolation and loneliness of ten associated with depression.

Conclusion:

Building resilience and coping skills is essential for healing and recovery from depression in children and adolescents. By teaching emotional regulation techniques, encouraging healthy lifestyle habits, and fostering positive relationships and peer support, young individuals can develop the tools and resources they need to navigate through depression and emerge stronger on the other side. It's important to provide a supportive environment where young individuals feel empowered to seek help, express their emotions, and engage in activities that promote their mental health and well-being. With the right support and guidance, children and adolescents can overcome depression and thrive in all aspects of their lives.

CHAPTER 7
ADDRESSING STIGMA AND MISCONCEPTION.

Stigma and misconceptions surrounding mental health can significantly impact the lives of young individuals struggling with depression. Addressing stigma and promoting mental health awareness are essential steps in creating supportive environments where children and adolescents feel safe seeking help and receiving the support they need. In this chapter, we will explore strategies for educating communities about youth depression and advocating for mental health awareness in schools and beyond.

Here are some strategies for educating communities about youth and children depression:

1. **Workshops and Presentations:** Organize workshops and presentations

in community centers, schools, and other public venues to provide information about youth and children depression. Invite mental health professionals, educators, and individuals with lived experience to share insights, dispel myths, and offer practical strategies for supporting young individuals.

2. **Informational Materials:** Create and distribute informational materials such as brochures, flyers, and posters that provide facts about youth depression, common symptoms, and available resources for support and treatment. Distribute these materials in schools, libraries, healthcare facilities, and community events to reach a wide audience.

3. **School-Based Programs:* * Collaborate with schools to implement mental health education programs that incorporate information about youth depression into the curriculum. Offer

training sessions for teachers and school staff on recognizing signs of depression in students and providing appropriate support and referrals to mental health services.

4. **Parent and Caregiver Workshops:** Host workshops and support groups specifically for parents and caregivers to discuss youth depression, its impact on children and adolescents, and effective strategies for supporting their mental health. Provide resources, guidance, and opportunities for parents to connect with each other and share experiences.

5. **Peer Education Programs:** Empower young individuals to become advocates for mental health by establishing peer education programs in schools and community organizations. Train peer leaders to facilitate discussions, organize events, and raise awareness about youth depression among their peers through presentations, activities, and social

media campaigns.

6. **Community Events:** Participate in community events such as health fairs, mental health awareness weeks, and youth summits to raise awareness about youth depression and promote positive mental health practices. Set up information booths, host interactive activities, and offer resources and referrals to support services.

7. **Collaboration with Healthcare Providers:** Partner with healthcare providers, including pediatricians, psychologists, and mental health clinics, to disseminate information about youth depression to patients and their families. Provide educational materials in waiting areas, offer training sessions for healthcare professionals, and establish referral networks for mental health services.

8. **Media Campaigns:** Utilize traditional and social media platforms

to launch awareness campaigns about youth depression. Develop engaging content such as videos, info graphics , and blog posts to share personal stories, provide education, and promote help-seeking behaviors among young individuals and their families.

9. **Cultural Sensitivity:** Recognize the importance of cultural sensitivity in educating communities about youth depression. Tailor educational materials and programs to address cultural beliefs, values, and barriers to seeking mental health support within diverse communities.

10. **Long-Term Engagement:** Foster long-term engagement and sustained efforts to educate communities about youth depression. Establish partnerships with local organizations, advocacy groups, and government agencies to coordinate ongoing initiatives, monitor progress, and evaluate the impact of educational

efforts over time.

Education is a powerful tool for dispelling myths and misinformation about youth depression. By providing accurate information about the causes, symptoms, and treatment options for depression, communities can better understand and support young

individuals experiencing mental health challenges.

Schools, community organizations, and healthcare providers can play a crucial role in educating parents, caregivers, teachers, and other stakeholders about youth depression. Workshops, presentations, and informational materials can help raise awareness and promote open discussions about mental health.

Moreover, incorporating mental health education into school curricula can help normalize conversations about mental health and reduce the stigma associated with seeking help. By teaching young individuals about the importance of mental health and well-being, communities can empower them to recognize when they or their peers may need support and where to turn for help.

Advocating for Mental Health Awareness in Schools and Beyond:

Advocacy efforts are essential for promoting mental health awareness and ensuring that young individuals receive the support and resources they need to thrive. Advocates can work to influence policies, allocate funding, and implement programs that prioritize mental health education and support services in schools and communities.

School-based mental health initiatives, such as counseling services, peer support groups, and mental health awareness campaigns, can help create a culture of support and acceptance within educational settings. By advocating for the integration of mental health education and resources into school policies and practices, advocates can help address stigma and promote early intervention for youth depression.

Beyond schools, advocacy efforts can focus on promoting mental health awareness in various community settings, including workplaces, healthcare facilities, and social service agencies. By collaborating with stakeholders from diverse sectors, advocates can raise awareness, reduce stigma, and improve access to mental health resources for young individuals and their families.

Conclusion:

Addressing stigma and misconceptions surrounding youth depression is essential for promoting mental health awareness and supporting young individuals in their journey towards healing and recovery. By educating communities about youth depression and advocating for mental health awareness in schools and beyond, we can create environments where children and adolescents feel empowered to seek help, receive support, and thrive. It's crucial to continue working together to break down barriers, challenge stigma, and promote understanding and acceptance of mental health issues among young individuals and the broader community.

CHAPTER 8.
SUPPORTING ACADEMIC SUCCESS AND WELL-BEING.

Academic success and social well-being are essential components of a child's development and overall mental health. For children and youths struggling with depression, it's crucial to implement strategies that support their academic achievement and foster positive social interactions. In this chapter, we will explore the importance of collaboration between schools, parents, and mental health professionals, as well as strategies for managing school-related stressors for children and youths dealing with depression.

Collaboration among Schools, mothers , and fathers, intellectual fitness experts, or Mental Health Professionals:

Effective collaboration between schools, parents, and mental health professionals is key to supporting children and youths with depression. By working together, these stakeholders can create a supportive environment that addresses the unique needs of each child and promotes their academic success and social well-being.

Schools can play a central role in facilitating collaboration by establishing open lines of communication with parents and providing access to mental health resources and support services within the school community. School counselors, psychologists, and different intellectual fitness experts and mental health workers can ideally labor closely with utmost carefulness and in collaboration with instructors, mothers and fathers, and parents to clearly pinpoint childrenand students battling or sufferingfrom depression, create and broaden individualized guide plans and support system, and monitor the positive effects over time.

Parents, on the other hand, can serve

as advocates for their children by actively participating in school meetings, sharing relevant information about their child's mental health history and treatment plan, and providing ongoing support and encouragement at home. By partnering with schools and mental health professionals, parents can help ensure that their child receives the necessary accommodations, interventions, and resources to thrive academically and socially.

Strategies for Managing School-related Stressors:

School-related stressors can exacerbate symptoms of depression in children and youths, making it challenging for them to focus on their academic responsibilities and engage in social activities. Implementing strategies to manage school-related stressors is essential for supporting their overall well-being and promoting resilience.

One effective strategy is to create a supportive and inclusive school environment where students feel valued, accepted, and understood. Schools can implement anti-bullying initiatives, promote diversity and inclusion, and provide opportunities for students to participate in extracurricular activities and peer support groups.

Additionally, schools can offer academic accommodations and support services to students with depression, such as flexible scheduling, homework extensions, and access to tutoring or academic counseling. By addressing academic challenges proactively, schools can help alleviate stress and promote academic success for children and youths struggling with depression.

Furthermore, teaching stress management and coping skills in schools can empower students to effectively manage school-related stressors and build resilience in the face of adversity. Techniques such as mindfulness, relaxation exercises, and time management strategies can help students develop healthy coping mechanisms and reduce the impact of stress on their mental health.

Supporting academic success and social well-being is essential for children and youths struggling with depression. By fostering collaboration between schools, parents, and mental health professionals, and implementing strategies for managing school-related stressors, we can create a supportive and nurturing environment where children and youths with depression can thrive academically and socially. It's essential to prioritize the holistic well-being of these individuals and provide them with the necessary support and resources to reach their full potential despite the challenges they may face.

CHAPTER 9.
PROMOTING A SENSE OF PURPOSE AND FULFILLMENT.

Promoting a Sense of Purpose and Fulfillment: Strategies for Children and Youths Struggling with Depression

Promoting a Sense of Purpose and Fulfillment.

Promoting a sense of purpose and fulfillment is crucial for children and youths struggling with depression. Finding meaning and enjoyment in life can enhance their resilience, improve their mental health, and contribute to their overall well-being. In this chapter, we will explore strategies for encouraging participation in hobbies and activities, as well as exploring opportunities for personal growth, to promote a sense of purpose and fulfillment for children and youths dealing with depression.

Encouraging Participation in Hobbies and Activities:

Engaging in hobbies and activities that bring joy and fulfillment can have a positive impact on a child's mental health and well-being. Encouraging children and youths to explore their interests, passions, and talents can provide them with a sense of purpose and accomplishment, which can help counteract the negative effects of depression.

Parents, caregivers, and educators can support children and youths in discovering and pursuing hobbies and activities that align with their interests and preferences. This may involve providing resources, guidance, and opportunities for exploration in various areas such as sports, arts and crafts, music, dance, gardening, or volunteer work.

Moreover, participating in hobbies and

activities can serve as a form of self-expression, stress relief, and social connection for children and youths struggling with depression. Engaging in enjoyable and meaningful activities can help distract from negative thoughts and emotions, boost self-esteem, and foster a sense of belonging and purpose within their communities.

Exploring Opportunities for Personal Growth:

Exploring opportunities for personal growth can empower children and youths to discover their strengths, develop new skills, and cultivate a sense of self-worth and confidence. Personal growth can occur through various avenues such as education, personal development workshops, mentoring programs, or challenging experiences that push individuals outside of their comfort zones.

Parents, educators, and mentors can

support children and youths in setting goals, overcoming obstacles, and embracing opportunities for personal growth and development. Encouraging them to step outside of their comfort zones, take on new challenges, and learn from setbacks can foster resilience and enhance their sense of agency and purpose.

Additionally, providing positive reinforcement, constructive feedback, and opportunities for reflection can help children and youths recognize their progress and accomplishments along their journey of personal growth. Celebrating their achievements and milestones can reinforce their sense of purpose and motivate them to continue striving for personal excellence despite the challenges they may face.

Promoting a sense of purpose and fulfillment is essential for children and youths struggling with depression. By encouraging participation in hobbies and activities and exploring opportunities for personal growth, we can empower them to find meaning, joy, and fulfillment in their lives. It's crucial to support their interests, passions, and aspirations, and provide them with the resources, guidance, and encouragement they need to thrive mentally, emotionally, and socially. With the right support and opportunities for growth, children and youths with depression can cultivate a sense of purpose and fulfillment that enriches their lives and contributes to their overall well-being.

CHAPTER 10.
NURTURING HOPE AND RECOVERY.

Strategies for Children and Yo uths Struggling with Depression

Nurturing hope and recovery is essential for children and youths struggling with depression. Instilling a sense of optimism and resilience can empower them to overcome challenges, navigate setbacks, and embark on a journey towards healing and recovery. In this chapter, we will explore strategies for celebrating progress and small victories, as well as emphasizing the importance of long-term support, in nurturing hope and recovery for children and youths dealing with depression.

some strategies for celebrating progress and small victories, nurturing hope and recovery for children and youths dealing with depression:

1. Acknowledge Achievements.

Take time to acknowledge and celebrate even the smallest achievements and progress made by children and youths struggling with depression. This could include completing a task, attending therapy sessions regularly, or expressing emotions in a healthy way. By recognizing their efforts, you validate their journey and boost their self-esteem.

2. Create a Celebration Ritual.

Establish a ritual for celebrating progress and small victories, such as having a weekly "achievement dinner" where the child gets to choose their favorite meal or a monthly "success party" where they receive small rewards or tokens of recognition for their accomplishments. Consistently celebrating their successes can create a positive atmosphere and reinforce their motivation to continue striving for recovery.

3. Use Positive Reinforcement.

Provide positive reinforcement through praise, encouragement, and affirmation whenever children and youths demonstrate resilience, effort, or progress in managing their depression symptoms. Positive reinforcement can help reinforce adaptive behaviors and build confidence in their ability to cope with challenges.

4. Set Realistic Goals.

Collaboratively set realistic and achievable goals with children and youths, taking into account their individual strengths, interests, and preferences. Break larger dreams and visions into smaller plausible steps, and rejoice in every milestone along the way. This approach helps to maintain motivation and momentum towards long-term recovery.

5. Encourage Self mirrored image or Reflection.

Encourage children and adolescents to reflect on their progress and identify areas of growth and improvement. Ask open-ended questions such as "What strategies have been helpful for you?" or "What challenges have you overcome recently?" Encouraging self mirrored image or reflection fosters self-awareness and empowers them to take an energetic function of their healingand recovery journey.

6. Provide Social Support.

Foster a supportive environment where children and youths feel validated and encouraged by their peers, family members, educators, and mental health professionals. Encourage friends and family to participate in celebrations and offer words of encouragement to the child. Social support reinforces their sense of belonging and strengthens their resilience in the face of challenges.

7. Normalize Setbacks:

Help children and youths understand that setbacks are a natural part of the recovery process and do not diminish their progress or potential for future success. Normalize setbacks by framing them as opportunities for learning and growth rather than failures. Emphasize resilience and perseverance as essential qualities for navigating through difficult times.

8. **Long-Term Support Planning:** Develop a comprehensive long-term support plan that addresses the ongoing needs of children and youths dealing with depression. This may involve regular check-ins with mental health professionals, participation in support groups or therapy sessions, and access to resources and coping strategies for managing future

challenges. Emphasize the importance of seeking help when needed and maintaining a support network thr oughout their recovery journey.

By implementing these strategies, caregivers, educators, and mental health professionals can create a nurturing environment that celebrates progress, reinforces resilience, and emphasizes the importance of long-term support in nurturing hope and recovery for children and y ouths dealing with depression.

Celebrating progress and small victories is an important part of nurturing hope and recovery for children and adolescent with depression. Acknowledging their efforts, achievements, and milestones can boost their self-esteem, reinforce positive behaviors, and provide motivation to continue moving forward despite obstacles.

Parents, caregivers, educators, and

mental health professionals can play a role in celebrating progress and small victories by providing praise, encouragement, and positive reinforcement. Whether it's completing a difficult task, reaching a personal goal, or demonstrating resilience in the face of adversity, recognizing and celebrating these accomplishments can foster a sense of pride and confidence in children and youths struggling with depression.

Moreover, celebrating progress and small victories can help shift the focus away from perceived failures or setbacks and highlight the progress that has been made along the journey of recovery. By reframing challenges as opportunities for growth and learning, children and youths can develop a more positive outlook on their abilities and potential for success.

Emphasizing the Importance of Long-Term Support:

Emphasizing the importance of long-term support is crucial for sustaining hope and recovery for children and youths with depression. Recovery is often a gradual and ongoing process that requires consistent support, encouragement, and resources over time.

Parents, caregivers, educators, and mental health professionals can work together to establish a supportive network of resources and services that address the diverse needs of children and youths struggling with depression. This may include access to counseling, therapy, medication management, peer support groups, and other mental health interventions.

Furthermore, fostering a sense of community and connection can provide children and youths with a support system that extends beyond their immediate circle of family and friends. Peer support groups, community organizations, and online forums can offer opportunities for social connection, validation, and shared experiences, which can be invaluable for maintaining hope and recovery in the long term.

Conclusion:

Nurturing hope and recovery is essential for children and youths struggling with depression. By celebrating progress and small victories and emphasizing the importance of long-term support, we can create a supportive environment where they feel empowered to overcome challenges, build resilience, and thrive despite their struggles. It's crucial to recognize and celebrate their achievements, no matter how small, and to provide ongoing support and encouragement as they continue on their journey of healing and recovery. With the proper resources, guidance, and support, young children and adolescents with depression can discover hope, resilience, and experience of motives or purpose that allows them to stay a satisfying and significant fulfilling, and meaningful lives.

EPILOGUE

As we close this guide on identifying depression in children and teenagers and providing strategies to help them recover quickly, it's essential to reflect on the journey we've taken together. Recognizing the signs of depression in young individuals is the first step towards supporting them on their path to healing and recovery.

We've explored the complexities of depression in the context of adolescence, understanding that it can manifest differently in each individual. By shedding light on the warning signs and symptoms, we've empowered caregivers, educators, and loved ones to intervene early and effectively.

Through a combination of professional support, compassionate listening, and fostering open communication, we've learned how to create a nurturing environment where teens and children feel safe to express their emotions and seek help without fear of judgment.

Remember, recovery is not a linear process, and setbacks may occur along the way. However, with patience, understanding, and a commitment to ongoing support, we can help our young ones navigate through the darkness of depression and emerge stronger, resilient, and equipped with the tools they need to thrive.Together, let's continue to advocate for mental health awareness and break the stigma surrounding depression, ensuring that every child and teenager receives the care and support they deserve on their journey towards healing and happiness.

AFTERWORD.

As we conclude this guide on identifying depression in children and teenagers and implementing strategies to aid in their speedy recovery, it's important to recognize that the journey towards mental wellness is ongoing. Our efforts to support young individuals struggling with depression extend far beyond the pages of this book. Each child and teenager battling depression is a unique individual with their own story, struggles, and strengths. While this guide provides a foundation for understanding and addressing depression, it is essential to remember that there is no one-size-fits-all solution. Flexibility, empathy, and adaptability are key as we navigate the complexities of mental health in young people.

We urge readers to continue educating themselves on mental health issues, fostering open dialogue within their communities, and advocating for accessible and comprehensive mental health resources for children and teenagers.

Together, let us strive to create a world where every child and teenager feels valued, supported, and empowered to seek help when needed. By working together, we can break the barriers surrounding depression and pave the way for a brighter, healthier future for our youth.

Acknowledgement:

My sincere acknowledgement to my mother who has always been a source of courage to me. My husband has been very supportive and encouraged me to put down my experiences as it will help many others.

About The Author

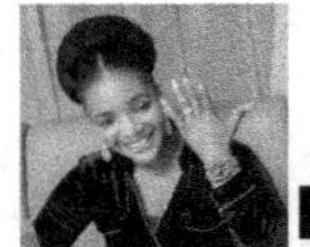

ELLIANA P. LEVI. Ph.D.

Is a health educationist. She holds a Ph.D.

in Health Management Science. A lecturer

at Urn Private University and Head Of the

Department of Faculty of Health Science at

the same University. Also a health

consultant St. Pricilla private clinic.

Praise For Author.

ELLIANA P. LEVI. **Ph.D.** is a dedicated health management scientist who does everything possible to get the best knowledge to serve her students and help clients with the best techniques for healthy living, healing, and recovery from different health challenges.

Attributes: Dedicated and devoted to her duties, friendly with both students and clients, lovely as she sees love as the first medicine for sick folks.